Contents

THE CHALLENGE OF CANCER

by

George Javor

Illness of any sort is a most unwelcome reminder of our frailty. But no sickness comes close to the devastating psychological impact of cancer. In fact, the typical reaction is one of incredulity: "This cannot be happening to me!" Instantly we seem to hear the sentence of death. Our perspective on existence undergoes rapid and drastic revision. The value of time increases immensely, while that of objects—"things"—depreciates markedly.

In a private survey by the ABC television company, Californians confessed to a greater dread of cancer than of being the victims of violent crimes or even of an atomic war. The diagnosis of cancer suddenly transforms an apparently healthy person to a seriously ill patient. It precipitates anxiety, anger, and grief.

Cover photo courtesy of the American Cancer Society

Southern Publishing Association, Nashville, Tennessee

Library of Congress Cataloging in Publication Data
Javor, George T 1940-
    The challenge of cancer.

    Bibliography: p. 96
    1. Cancer. 2. Christian life—1960-
I. Title. [DNLM: 1. Neoplasms—Popular works.
QZ201 J41c]
RC263.J38   616.99'4   79-29674
ISBN 0-8127-0275-1

Preface

Practically every day we read about cancer in the newspapers, but our understanding of the subject has not increased greatly. Conflicting theories, extravagant claims, optimistic predictions, and depressing statistics constantly confront us. Cancer has so many facets that it is not possible to embrace its totality in an article.

At the same time we no longer have a choice as to whether we want to know more about cancer or not. It affects so many of us one way or another that each one of us must learn a few pertinent facts about it. At the minimum, we should know the meaning of the term "cancer," some of the disease's causes, how it is treated, and what we can do to prevent it. We also must put ourselves into the shoes of those afflicted with the illness so that we may meet their needs more adequately. I wrote this small book in an attempt to meet the challenge of knowing as much as possible about cancer. The reader can obtain more information from the sources cited in the bibliography. It is my hope that by becoming more familiar with it the reader will lose some of the dread of cancer.

Chapter 1

The Scope of Cancer

Like it or not, cancer affects everyone. Statisticians assure us that the odds are one in four that we shall contract it. If we don't, we will have close relatives and friends who will.

Cancer most commonly strikes in the latter third of our "threescore and ten" years. Indeed, a direct correlation exists between cancer mortality and age. However, this does not guarantee immunity to younger people, for cancer is no respecter of age.

Many regard cancer in a fatalistic light, that is, it strikes unpredictably and that we can do little to prevent it. However, it is becoming increasingly apparent that this is not the case. Far from being unpredictable, certain types of cancers now have clearly identifiable causes.

Cancer is as old as recorded history. The

earliest records of India, Greece, and Egypt mention tumors. The Greeks called the disease *karkinos* (crab), because of the clawlike appearance of spreading cancers. The Romans translated the Greek *karkinos* to the Latin "cancer," and the word filtered into our modern English usage.

The number of deaths from cancer is on the rise. Partly this has resulted because medical science has eliminated infectious diseases as a major cause of death, and an increased number of individuals live into their sixties and seventies. The other contributing factor is our modern style of living.

Each year physicians diagnose more than 600,000 new cases of cancer in the United States alone. The second leading killer in this country, it results in more than 300,000 deaths in a year. For children between the ages one through fourteen it is the largest single cause of death. In terms of loss of working life, cancer destroys each year more than a million and a half man-years.

In 1970 a special panel of consultants assembled by the U.S. Senate published a report entitled "A National Program for the Conquest of Cancer." The report indicates that cancer is the primary health concern of the people of the United States. In numerous polls about two thirds of those questioned admitted a greater dread of cancer than of any other illness.

The report also made some interesting observations on funds for cancer research. The 1969 budget allowed 89 cents a person toward the effort. At the same time we had allocated $19 a person for foreign aid and the space program, $125 a person for the war in Vietnam, and $410 for national defense. In the same year, deaths from cancer were five and a half times the number of casualties from car accidents, and also more than all American servicemen killed in World War II.

Not all tumors are synonymous with *cancer*. Those growths that do not invade neighboring tissues, but remain localized, scientists call benign tumors. Cancer refers to the kind of uncontrolled growth that spreads from the tissue of origin to other parts of the body. It is a catchword for four main types of growths: the carcinomas, sarcomas, leukemias, and lymphomas.

If the growth originates in the epithelia (the sheets of cells covering the body), the cancer is a "carcinoma." More than 90 percent of cancers are carcinomas. When the tissue of origin is in the fibrous muscle tissue, bone, or in the blood vessels, we are dealing with "sarcoma." "Leukemias" arise in the blood-forming tissue of the bone marrow, and "lymphomas" in the lymph nodes.

The usual classification of cancer is by the organ it originally affected. Based on this, medical science recognizes about two hundred different varieties. It is useful to catalog such growths by the organ of origin because each type appears to result from different causes. Eliminating the cause for one kind does not readily alter the incidence of other types.

Many of the two hundred types of cancers are rare. The most frequent varieties involve a much smaller number. Ten types of cancers—those of the colon and rectum, breast, lung and bronchus, prostate, uterus, lymph organs, bladder, stomach, blood, and pancreas—account for three quarters of all malignancies.

In the forest of technical terms and statistics, it is easy to lose sight of the individual afflicted with cancer. In the following pages, after discussing the nature of cancer, its causes and cures, we will consider the needs of the person battling the illness.

Chapter 2

Of Growing

All living matter possesses the capacity for growth. Only by growth can the fertilized eggs of higher organisms become adult forms. The early stages of embryonic growth frequently occur at a phenomenal speed, but during the later development of the organism the rates gradually diminish. By adult life some organs, such as the brain, have altogether lost their capacity to regenerate.

Most organs, nevertheless, retain their ability to grow by cell division. The cells of the inner lining of the intestines grow and divide quite rapidly, but the same tissues also have a high rate of cell loss. Skin cells ordinarily divide slowly, but during wound healing they speed up.

The process by which cells proliferate is

complex and we do not completely understand it. Before cell division can take place, the cell manufactures thousands of substances within it so that identical copies of all components can end up in both "daughter cells." The time of preparation for cell division varies among tissues from hours to days.

The single most important cellular components are the chromosomes, found within the nucleus of the cell. Chromosomes contain deoxyribonucleic acid (DNA) molecules, which bear the genetic information. The nuclei of cells and the chromosomes within them are invisible to the naked eye, but if one could stretch out end to end the DNA molecules packaged in a single nucleus, they would span an unbelievable six feet.

These extraordinarily long molecules carry all necessary instructions for the manufacture of new cellular components. Higher organisms, such as ourselves, consist of numerous types of specialized cells. Our organs—the eyes, kidneys, heart, liver, bones—function properly because of the unique capabilities of their individual cells. The genetic material, the DNA molecules, direct the formation of such specialized cells.

Of Growing

Each cell in our body with a nucleus contains the identical type of genetic material. It follows, then, that not every cell uses all of the available genetic information. If it did, all cells would be identical.

The information content of DNA molecules is arranged into small units called genes. "Structural" genes direct the manufacture of the thousands of different protein and ribonucleic acid molecules that operate the cell's machinery. "Regulatory" genes control the activities of the structural genes. During embryonic development the thousands of structural and regulatory genes click on and off in a predetermined order, producing specialized cells.

Cancer cells are, however, unique in the way they divide. Frequently their daughter cells are not identical, as we can easily tell by counting the chromosomes of cancer cells. They usually possess fewer, though sometimes more, chromosomes than normal cells. (For humans, the usual number is forty-six.) Moreover, the shapes of the cancer cell's chromosomes are frequently abnormal as well. Not surprisingly, therefore, cancer cells usually suffer from deficiencies, imbalances, and other irregularities.

Many believe that cancer cells develop rapidly. In fact, cancer cells are quite sick, and most of the time they do not grow as well as healthy ones. The only reason that cancerous tumors overwhelm healthy tissue is lack of growth on the part of normal cells.

Regular cells are sensitive to what scientists call contact inhibition. When the boundary of such a cell touches the outer surface of neighboring identical cells, growth automatically ceases in that direction. Cancer cells, in contrast, are insensitive to contact. Tissue cultures of healthy and cancerous cells will graphically show this. The healthy cells proliferate on top of the nutrient medium until they form a solid, single layer of tissue. Cancer cells, on the other hand, spread in a haphazard manner, creating a disorderly, misshapen mass until they run out of nutrients.

Evidence suggests that healthy cells can divide only a predetermined number of times. Then the cell dies. This accounts for the mystery of aging, as systematic deterioration of tissues and organs occur. Strangely, cancer cells do not have this limitation. Hela cells, a frequently used line of cancer cells, for instance, originated in a woman who died of cancer some thirty years ago. Thus, when normal cells transform into cancer cells, they achieve a potential for "immortality," a dubious honor, to be sure.

Continuous, unrelenting growth and cell division have truly dramatic consequences. If we imagine a typical cell, which divides once in twenty-four hours, we can estimate the increase of cellular volume with the passage of time. A single cell occupies the tiny space of 10,000-millionth of a cubic inch, visible only under a good-quality microscope. After twenty days, however, the cellular mass is already visible. It is about the size of a pinhead. Another ten days of growth, and it is a small cube, like half a small pair of dice. Forty days from the beginning of our experiment we have a quart of cells. In another ten days, it totals 250 gallons. If it continued seventy more days, the cellular growth would be the size of the earth.

It may appear that the cellular mass has exploded in size. But in fact the rate of growth is constant, and the dramatic increases in size come about as a normal consequence of exponential growth (continuous doubling of every cell). The trouble with cancer cells is not that they grow but that they do so in an uncontrolled manner, and thus they block and displace healthy tissue.

Applying this principle to leukemic cell growth leads us to the following observations (blood cells happen to grow, not in clumps, but diffusedly in the bone marrow, which normally contains more than one million million—10^{12}—normal cells): If it takes a week for the leukemic cells to double their number, then it requires thirty weeks before one billion cancer cells are present in the bone marrow. At this stage they comprise only a thousandth of the normal cell population and, as such, remain undetectable. Another five weeks increases the leukemic cell number to about 5 percent of the normal cells. Now we can diagnose the disease. However, cancer cells by now have undergone thirty-five divisions, and if permitted to continue for another five to seven more doublings, they kill the patient.

Present treatments aim at reducing the number of leukemic cells in the patient's body so that the normal ones can continue to function. We have no means at present to totally eradicate such a large population of leukemic cells.

Chapter 3

What Causes Cancer?

Cancer is perhaps the only current disease induced by a multitude of agents, yet whose immediate cause remains unknown. Chemical substances, biological agents, radiation, and physical irritation can initiate it. Because of the bewildering array and lack of a common bond between the various agents, some researchers have suggested that cancer is a collective term for a host of diverse diseases. However, the majority view among scientists at present is that all cancer-causing agents (carcinogens) somehow modify the chromosomes of their target cells, which acts as the underlying factor behind cancer. Such a generalization is helpful but not as enlightening as it may sound. In reality, we have not identified the critical molecular change in any type of cancer.

Scientists call the substances that alter the genetic material, DNA, mutagens. They envision that some mutagens chemically modify portions of the DNA molecules of the chromosomes, altering their information contents. Other potentially harmful substances induce the cellular machinery to miscopy the genetic material. Nucleic acids from viruses, too, can act as mutagens when they attach to their host's genetic apparatus. Moreover, certain forms of radiation may physically damage the chromosomes.

Most alternations of the genetic material are permanent in the sense that the changes pass from one generation to the next. Since chromosomes can get modified in many different ways, it is not surprising to find so many diverse processes that lead to cancer.

To be sure, not every mutation-causing substance is carcinogenic, and neither are all known carcinogens mutagens as well. However, the exceptions form only a small minority.

Chemical Carcinogens
The actual number of documented human

chemical hazards is small. It comprises a handful of compounds to which industrial workers were exposed at extraordinarily high concentrations, a few drugs, and the contents of cigarette smoke. Table 1 lists the substances:

Table 1:
Chemicals known to be carcinogenic to man

> aflatoxin
> auramine (the manufacturing process of this dye)
> benzene
> benzidine
> bis (chloromethyl) ether
> cadmium oxide
> chloramphenicol
> chromium
> cyclophosphamide
> diethylstilbesterol
> hematite (the mining process of this substance)
> melphalan
> mustard gas
> 2-naphthylamine
> nickel

N, N-bis (-2-chloroethyl)
    2-naphthylamine
N, N-bis (-2-chloroethyl) . . . etc.
soot, tars, and oils
vinyl chloride

The reader can readily understand that testing suspected carcinogenic materials in humans is a most difficult undertaking. Researchers face numerous complicating factors such as the impossibility of controlling the diets and activities of the test subjects for years at a time, the lack of adequate numbers of test subjects, and the long latent periods of many carcinogens. For example, the tars of tobacco smoke cause lung cancer typically after a period of twenty years.

Further complications arise from the discovery of substances not in themselves dangerous but which enhance the effectiveness of carcinogens. Such materials, called promotors, or cocarcinogens, can increase the carcinogenic potential of a substance manyfold. Low doses of polycyclic hydrocarbons and nitrosamines represent one such combination. When administered singly, neither causes lung cancer in rats or mice, but the two agents together produce cancer in a significant number of animals. It so happens that cigarette smoke contains both types of chemicals.

Some evidence indicates that compounds causing cancers in animals are also potentially carcinogenic in humans. In the early 1940s researchers reported that a substance named diethylstilbesterol produces tumors in animals. Nevertheless, in the 1950s it became a popular drug for the prevention of natural abortions. Only in 1971 did its carcinogenic activity in humans come to light. Then new studies showed that cancer of the cervix resulted in those daughters whose mothers had used the drug during their pregnancies.

As useful as animal testing for carcinogenicity is, it is a costly and time-consuming process. A conservative estimate places $250,000 and three years of time for the proper evaluation of a single substance. Thus far scientists have examined about 7,000 chemicals for carcinogenicity in animals and have found a little more than 1,500 that cause cancer. Not all reported tests on animals were scientifically correct. The approximate number of carcinogens established by this method therefore is small, maybe two thirds to one half of what is reported.

Animal studies have indicated several classes of chemicals to be carcinogenic. They include synthetic organic substances, naturally occurring compounds, and inorganic substances.

Among the synthetic organic carcinogens, the first ones discovered in the 1930s were the polycyclic aromatic hydrocarbons. The most powerful is benzopyrene, a component of coal tar. Workers in industries using coal tar contracted skin cancer in unusually high numbers, which tipped off epidemiologists (those who study epidemic diseases) of its dangers.

Benzopyrene is the main hydrocarbon carcinogen in cigarette smoke. When applied to the skin of a mouse twice weekly for seven weeks it causes a benign tumor to appear on that spot. If one stops the carcinogen treatment, the skin will reabsorb the tumor, and it disappears. However, if the skin is exposed to benzopyrene for four more weeks, the tumor turns malignant and eventually kills the animal. Orally administered, the hydocarbon causes malignancy of the mammary glands, of the lungs, and of the blood-forming tissues of mice.

Benzopyrene has turned up in a wide variety of substances, including lubricating machine oils, exhaust fumes of internal-combustion engines, charcoal-broiled steaks, roasted coffee and chickory, smoked sausage, charred dough, caramelized sugar, and French fries.

Another class of organic carcinogens is the aromatic amines. The manufacture of certain textile dyes before 1960 extensively employed benzidine and 2-naphthylamine. Then scientists discovered their carcinogenic properties. 4-dimethylaminoazobenzene was used to color butter and oil up to around 1935, when researchers found it generated cancer of the liver or skin in mice and rats.

A third group of organic carcinogens consists of different types of substances, including sulfur mustards used as poison gas in World War I, commonly used industrial solvents—dioxane and carbon tetrachloride—the insecticides—DDT, aldrin, endrin—and polychlorinated biphenyls (PCBs), used as additives in plastics manufacture. In addition, there is vinyl chloride, the starting compound for the manufacture of polyvinyl chloride and, until recently, the propellant gas in spray cans.

The last class of organics that cause cancer in animals is the nitrosamines. Of 200 nitrosamines tested, 180 were carcinogenic. Nitrosamines easily form from secondary amines and nitrous acid, or from amines and nitrogen oxide of the air in the presence of strong light. Not surprisingly, then, scientists have detected them in polluted air, in processed fish, in certain cheeses, and in cured ham and fried bacon. Because most processed meats contain some sodium nitrite as an additive and secondary amines are present naturally, nitrosamines can form in the acid environment of the stomach during digestion.

That some man-made synthetics are carcinogenic is easier to accept than the startling fact that carcinogens occur in nature as well. Some of the natural substances have only weak activity, while others are extremely potent carcinogens. Aflatoxin B1, produced by the yellow mold, *Aspergillus flavus*, is among the most powerful carcinogens known. A single injection of ten-millionth of a gram under the skin of a mouse causes sarcoma. *Aspergillus* often contaminates peanuts. Safrole, present in sassafras, capsaicin in chili peppers, and parasorbic acid in mountain ash berries represent but a few of the substances that show carcinogenic acitivity in animal testing.

As a precautionary measure, it is wise to avoid foods produced by molds such as certain cheeses, exotic spices, and herbs. Most likely the above-listed substances represent only the tip of the iceberg. With time, we can expect that science will uncover numerous carcinogens among other items in our current diet.

All processed foods found on grocery shelves contain numerous additives. Such substances enhance the flavor, appearance, and shelf life of the product. All food additives receive thorough testing and must be licensed for use. What the laboratories do not check, however, is what happens when the individual subjects a variety of additives to baking temperatures. At 450°F two chemicals may easily recombine to produce new unsuspected materials, which could be potentially harmful. It is a sad fact that we just do not know much about the chemical changes that occur in foods at baking temperatures.

Another, yet different, class of potential carcinogens consists of inorganic metals and minerals. Beryllium salts produced cancer of the lungs in monkeys. Evidence also exists for the carcinogenic nature of cadmium, chromium, cobalt, nickel, and lead powders. Arsenic provokes cancer of the respiratory tract in humans. Asbestos forms thin microscopic needles that can accumulate in certain parts of living cells. It causes mesotheliomas, cancers that originate from the epithelium lining of internal body cavities.

Each year technology introduces nearly a thousand new chemicals to the public, and the number of substances yet untested for carcinogenic activity runs into the millions. There are not enough toxicologists, pathologists, laboratory facilities, animal suppliers, and financial resources to examine all known chemicals. A recent estimate puts the total global capacity of scientists to adequately test for carcinogenicity, using animals, to six hundred substances a year.

Scientists have searched for structural similarities among the known carcinogens, hoping to find a way to predict the sinister potential among yet untested substances. Their efforts have met with some success. They now recognize that most chemical carcinogens are strong electrophilic substances. ("Electrophilic" is a term chemists employ to describe compounds that seek out other substances rich in electrons and become bound to them.) As interesting and potentially useful as the observation is, it is still not specific enough to predict whether a given compound will be carcinogenic. There are simply too many electrophilic substances that are harmless as far as cancer is concerned.

Another generalization, mentioned earlier, is that almost all carcinogens are also mutagens. That fact is the basis of a rapid, inexpensive method to test for potential carcinogens developed by Bruce Ames of the University of California at Berkeley. It uses mutant strains of the bacterium *Salmonella typhimurium*, which cannot grow without the amino acid, histidine.

The test runs in the following manner: The researcher places about a billion bacterial cells on top of an agar surface and mixes them with the compound he wishes to test. He also adds a small amount of rat liver homogenate to the mixture. If the material is a mutagen, it causes random changes in the genes of the bacteria and some of the new alterations may correct the original mutation. Such cells can grow once again in the absence of the amino acid, histidine, and form visible colonies on the agar surface. The more powerful the mutagen, the more numerous the bacterial colonies.

The liver homogenate converts potentially dangerous substances to the active form of the mutagen. Medical science now recognizes that many cancer-causing substances are quite harmless in the form we ingest or inhale them. But our enzymes, especially those of the liver, convert them to their active, harmful form.

In one set of experiments, out of 175 different known carcinogens tested by the technique, 157, or 90 percent, were mutagenic. Similarly, when researchers examined known nonmutagenic materials, 94 out of 108, or 87 percent, behaved as expected. The "Ames" test gave the first indications that certain hair dyes and Tris, the flame retardant used in children's pajamas, were potential cancer hazards. Since then, animal tests have proved them carcinogenic.

At least a thousand industrial, government, and academic laboratories throughout the world routinely use the test. It costs $300 to $1,000 for each chemical studied and yields results in weeks.

The Ames test, however, is not uniformly

reliable for all types of substances. Antimetabolites, polychlorinated cyclic compounds, and steroids, among others, do not correlate well with the results of long-term animal studies. Apparently most substances that undergo complex changes during digestion or other metabolic processes also fall in this category.

Therefore, researchers are developing other short-term tests to complement it. They employ other microorganisms, the fruit fly Drosophila, and cultured mammalian cells. The lab can examine a potential carcinogenic substance with a battery of short-term tests, and hopefully their combined results will correlate well with carcinogenic activity in animals.

Viruses

Viruses are minuscule parasites, preying on every known form of life. Incapable of living by themselves, they are merely complexes of nucleic acids and proteins. Neither do they have any known useful function, and if viruses ceased to exist, the plant and animal world would escape a multitude of diseases.

They range in size from a millionth of a

millimeter to 250 times that size, and they are visible only under the electron microscope. Viruses have varied shapes, from round to polygonal.

The surfaces of all viruses consist of proteins, and inside are their infective material, either deoxyribonucleic acids (DNA) or ribonucleic acids (RNA), but never both. Thus we speak of DNA or RNA containing viruses.

The proteins protect the viral nucleic acids and contain binding sites to specific target cells of their host. Each virus infects only certain types of organisms. Plants, microorganisms, insects, mammals, birds, fish—all play host to a select group of viruses.

Viruses attach themselves to their host and either inject their nucleic acid into a cell or allow the host to engulf them and digest their protein coats. In either case the viral nucleic acids find their way into the host cell.

Once inside, the viral nucleic acids begin using the cell's elaborate machinery to their own end. They shut down the host's control system and take over operation of the cell. It is as if a foreign army invaded a certain country, and after capturing the vital control centers, it used the country's own civil-service structure to their own ends.

Soon after the virus infects the cell, one can detect multitudes of virus particles inside it. Eventually there are so many particles that the cell bursts, releasing hundreds of newly made viruses to the neighboring cells. The process then repeats itself until it has destroyed a whole section of tissue.

Occasionally, however, viral infection can follow a different pattern. Here the viral nucleic acids simply attach themselves to the host's own genetic material and remain inactive. When the host cell duplicates its own genes, the attached viral nucleic acid is copied too. The additional piece of viral genetic substance may or may not alter the cell's characteristics. In some cases researchers find merely a few new proteins in the cell. But in other instances the cell undergoes a "transformation" from a normal to a malignant type.

Scientists have firmly established that some viruses—called oncogenic viruses— cause cancers in animals. The first known virus-induced cancer was chicken leukosis, investigated by Ellerman and Bang in 1908. A few years later Rous found that one could transmit sarcomas in Plymouth Rock hens by extracts of the cancerous tissue previously passed through filters to remove any bacteria. During the early 1930s Richard Shope described viruses that caused warts and skin cancers in rabbits. Later in the same decade Bittner found evidence for the viral origin of breast cancers in certain strains of mice. In 1951 Gross wrote of the production of leukemia in a certain strain of mice. The researchers injected them when one day old with cell-free extracts of leukemia arising in another strain of mice. Later experiments showed that even if one induced the leukemia in mice by radiation, they could transmit it to other mice with the use of cell-free extracts. It seems that irradiation activated some dormant, potentially oncogenic virus in mice.

Human polio virus generates cancer when injected into young specimens of lower animals: guinea pigs, rabbits, rats, and ferrets. Adenoviruses 12 and 18, which cause minor respiratory illnesses in man, such as sore throats and slight colds, induce cancers in newborn hamsters. A monkey virus, SV40, can transform tissue cultures of healthy human embryo cells to malignant ones. All in all, scientists have discovered more than one hundred different strains of animal tumor viruses. Vaccines prepared against specific oncogenic viruses reduced the cancer rate among exposed animals.

Scientists strongly suspect that viruses have a part to play in certain human cancers. Current research is zeroing in on the role of certain RNA viruses, the B and C types, in cancers of the breast and certain sarcomas. Among DNA viruses, some of the herpes viruses, such as the herpes simplex type II in cervical carcinoma and the Epstein-Barr virus in Burkitt's lymphoma and Hodgkin's disease appear to have a causative role. But despite suspicions, researchers have not pinpointed a human oncogenic virus. Once they identify such an agent, they can prepare a vaccine which would protect individuals from that type of a cancer.

It is noteworthy that in animal studies almost always the viruses induce the cancers in young specimens whose immunologic defense mechanism has not yet developed. The inescapable conclusion is that the host's immune defense mechanism manages to cope, under normal circumstances, with the onslaught of oncogenic viruses.

In humans, if viruses alone could produce cancers, we would expect cancer epidemics, much like other virus-caused diseases such as smallpox, measles, mumps. But that is not generally the case. Researchers have found a clustering of occurrences in the case of Burkitt lymphoma. However, it appears that in addition to infection by the Epstein-Barr virus, other factors also contribute to the development of the disease, including the specific genetic background, heavy malarial exposure, and other yet unidentified environmental factors. Incidences of tumors of certain organs have variations of 100- to 200-fold, depending on the geographic location. This suggests that environmental causes are important. Leukemia and lymphoma cases, on the other hand, appear more uniformly around the world, which could indicate viruses as a causal agent. RNA-containing virus indicators have turned up in leukemias, sarcomas, and breast carcinomas, but researchers have not yet observed complete virus particles.

Radiation

"Radiation" is a term that describes waves of various types of energy traveling through space. (Some forms of radiation may also contain tiny pieces of matter.) We are grateful for the low-energy waves of light, heat, and sound as they crisscross our paths and bounce into us constantly. Radio and television waves are also of the low-energy type, and as such, they are physiologically harmless.

Exposure to high-energy radiation, on the other hand, is potentially dangerous. The ultraviolet rays of the sun, X rays generated by high-voltage instruments, and gamma rays emanating from certain radioactive elements can threaten one's health.

High-energy radiation penetrates most biologic tissue and generates ions in its path. Ions are positively or negatively charged particles. Some of them may cause unusual and undesirable chemical changes in the organism.

Laboratory studies on animals have produced evidence that high-energy radiation causes cancer. Increased doses of X rays resulted in a corresponding increase in myeloid leukemia in male RF-type mice. Sprague-Dawley strain in female rats developed breast tumors within one year after X-ray irradiation, again in proportion to the dosage received. By

using varying amounts of radiation, researchers could cause cancers on any part of an organism.

A similar situation exists for humans. The
data are not as extensive as with animal
studies, but they are conclusive enough.
Workers freely exposed to radioactive substances before science realized the harmful
side effects, survivors of the atomic bombs of
Hiroshima and Nagasaki, and patients ir-
radiated for diagnostic or therapeutic purposes have all shown notable increases in the
various leukemias, cancers of the female
breast, of the thyroid gland, of lymphoid tissues, of the bronchus, and of the gastrointestinal tract.

Cancer does not immediately appear after
irradiation. Prenatal exposure to high-energy
radiation can lead to juvenile leukemias and
solid tumors within two or three years after
birth, reaching their peak in the fifth year.
Only after eight years does the cancer risk become insignificant. Exposure to high-energy
radiation after birth can have a latent period of
a decade or more before solid tumors appear. It
is also possible that some exposures to radiation carry an increased risk of cancer for the

rest of the life, for science has recorded latent periods as long as thirty to forty years.

Ultraviolet rays are the most common type of high-energy radiation reaching us. They primarily affect the skin, and excessive amounts lead to skin cancer. Caucasians who spend more time outdoors are more likely to develop skin cancer. In such cases, cancer is most frequent on the unclothed areas of the body. The extent of exposure to ultraviolet radiation depends on the geographic location as well as on the life-style.

Ultraviolet rays damage the genetic material of the skin cells. To be sure, such cells have a certain amount of ability to repair radiation damage. Interestingly, visible light activates the repair mechanism. However excessive exposures defeat it. Individuals with the inherited condition called xeroderma pigmentosum lack this repair mechanism and, as a consequence, almost always develop skin cancer.

A thin ozone layer that shields us from the most energetic types of solar ultraviolet radiation surrounds our earth's atmosphere. Ozone is a gas, composed of a form of oxygen and recognizable by its unpleasant, sharp odor. Engines of high-flying supersonic airplanes routinely burn up small portions of the earth's ozone layer. Fortunately ozone is continually produced in the upper atmosphere, and over a period of time the loss can be replenished. However, if the number of supersonic flights increases, we could face a gradual depletion of ozone.

Some man-made pollutants such as chloro-fluoromethane, used as aerosol propellants, refrigerants, and industrial cleaners also destroy ozone when carried to the upper atmosphere by air currents. A 10 percent reduction in the ozone layer will increase our exposure to ultraviolet radiation by 20 percent so that the incidence of skin cancer would rise 142 percent in Dallas, Texas, and 62 percent in St. Paul, Minnesota.

Physical Irritants

Various plastics such as Bakelite, cellophane, polyethylene, polyvinyl chloride, Dacron, nylon, polystyrene, even stainless-steel films when implanted into rats, produce sarcomas. Such substances cannot enter into chemical reactions, and therefore we conclude that their carcinogenicity arises from their long-term irritation of the tissue.

Among stomach-cancer patients we commonly find that stomach ulcers or long-standing mucosal inflammation precedes the malignancy. Primary cancer of the liver frequently occurs in regions where cirrhosis was present. Cancer also often follows severe burns or ulcer scars. Gallbladder cancers frequently develop from the chronic irritation of gallstones.

It is difficult to see how irritating substances can alter the genetic material enough to transform healthy cells into cancerous ones. One view is that physical irritants are not really carcinogens themselves but are highly effective cocarcinogens, that is, agents that promote the development of cancer in conjunction with something else.

Heredity

Environmental factors cause an estimated 80 percent of cancer. Chemicals, viruses, radiation, and physical irritation all belong to this category. However, evidence indicates that heredity, too, plays a role in the development of cancer.

An experimentally developed, highly inbred strain of mice (strain AKR), for instance, has a much higher rate of spontaneous tumor formation than other strains. Similarly, the B-6 strain is much more sensitive to hydrocarbon-induced cancer than the other varieties of laboratory mice. In both cases the increased susceptibilities have a genetic origin.

Among humans, scientists have identified genetic factors in certain rare forms of cancer, such as xeroderma pigmentosum (which leads to skin cancer), retinoblastoma (a cancer of the eye), Gardner's syndrome (polyps in the colon), to mention a few.

Studies on the movement of populations help us detect environmental and genetic factors in cancer development. Rates of stomach cancers in Japan are high compared to the United States, but those of cancers of the large intestine, breasts, and prostate are much less frequent. When Japanese emigrate to the United States the differences in the rates of stomach, large intestine, and prostate cancers disappear within two generations, even though Japanese immigrants tend to inter-marry. Breast cancers, on the other hand, continue to be of low incidence among Japanese women. Such observations implicate the environment as a major factor in the first three cancers and as a genetic element for cancer of the breast.

Indeed, other studies support this conclusion. Among the common types of cancers, susceptibility to breast cancer has the strongest correlation with genetic background. But researchers have made studies on the clustering in families of cancers of the colon and bronchus as well. A two- to three-fold increase in colon cancer occurs among close relatives, and individuals who both smoked and had a blood relative suffering from lung cancer had a fourteenfold increased risk of contracting the same illness.

As we pointed out earlier, the enzymes of the body modify most chemical carcinogens into their "active" form. Individuals vary greatly in the levels of their enzymes. Therefore, one who happens to have a high level of an activating enzyme would be more prone to contract a certain type of cancer than someone else with a lower level. Since genes regulate enzyme production, then one's susceptibility or resistance to cancer partially depends on heredity.

For example, numerous studies on the role of benzopyrene in human lung cancer point to wide differences among individuals in their susceptibility to the pollutant. (Benzopyrene occurs in cigarette smoke, polluted air, and barbecued meat.) At least three enzymes alter the carcinogen in the body. One of them is the Aryl hydrocarbon hydroxylase, AHH, which converts the carbon-carbon double bonds of benzopyrene to epoxides (two carbon atoms attached to an oxygen atom).

Scientists consider the newly made epoxides to be the real carcinogens, as they can react directly with the genetic apparatus of the cell. Studies showed that genes controlled the level of the AHH enzyme. Among healthy individuals, 42.2 percent had low AHH activity and 57.8 percent had intermediate or high-enzyme activities. But among patients with lung cancer 5 percent had low AHH activity and 95 percent had intermediate or high AHH activity.

The data suggests that individual susceptibility to cancers varies according to genetic factors. (We assume here that smoking itself does not raise the level of AHH.)

Chapter 4

An Ounce of Prevention

At the conclusion of the Cold Spring Harbor symposium on the origins of human cancer, in September, 1976, Dr. J. Cairns of the Imperial Cancer Research Fund, London, England, made some incisive comments. He observed that during the second half of the nineteenth century, mortality from bacterial diseases had dropped in Western countries by almost tenfold (that is, eliminating nine out of ten deaths) through improvements in public health and preventive medicine. In terms of the number of lives saved, such steps were of far greater consequence than the subsequent discovery of antibiotics. The lesson is clear for the attack on cancer. Prevention is probably a more effective (though less spectacular) means of saving people from death by cancer than any actual cure that may come some time in the future.

To prevent cancer will be far more complicated than were the successful measures taken against bacterial infections because of the great diversity of cancer-causing agents. The task of identifying carcinogens and cocarcinogens has merely begun. Yet a 1975 report, using current knowledge of carcinogenesis, projected that already we could have avoided 30 percent of the estimated deaths from cancer during the next year (see Table 2 for details). This indeed is encouraging.

Researchers estimate that environmental factors either cause outright, or at least stimulate, a full 80 percent of all cancers. If their guess is correct, then future efforts to uncover environmental carcinogens could lead to the elimination of eight out of ten deaths.

Naturally, to benefit from such research, we will have to alter our life-styles, diet, and environment. While in theory it is self-evident, it has not worked too well in practice. It seems that for many the threat of cancer is not a sufficiently powerful force to change ingrained habits.

A good example in the United States is the

An Ounce of Prevention

Table 2:
Preventable Cancer Deaths
From *Prevention and Detection of Cancer*, H. E. Nieburgs, ed.
(Marcel Dekker, Inc.), 1978, p. 871.

1. Mortality reducible through lowered exposure

Cancer Sites	Preventable Contributing Factors:	1976 Deaths in U.S. Expected	Preventable
lung, larynx, other respiratory	cigarette smoking, occupational exposures, urban pollutants	88,000	72,000
oral cavity, head, neck, esophagus	cigarette smoking, high alcohol intake	15,000	7,100
bladder, liver	cigarette smoking, industrial exposure, alcohol	19,000	8,300
pancreas	cigarette smoking	19,000	6,300
colon, rectum	aspects of diet, high fat intake, low bulk	50,000	14,000
breast	aspects of diet, high fat intake, low bulk	33,000	9,400
skin (melanoma and other)	sunlight, some industrial exposure	5,000	1,200

2. Mortality reducible through earlier diagnosis and treatment

breast	screening	33,000	3,300
uterine cervix	screening	7,700	1,500

high number of cigarette smokers despite the undeniably harsh consequences of their habit. The Surgeon General first warned the smoking public in 1964 after a careful survey of the data from 6,000 research reports. In 1978 the Surgeon General issued a second warning summarizing more than 25,000 scientific papers. It repeated the same message even more emphatically, linking not only many cancers with smoking but various heart ailments as well. The Secretary of Health, Education, and Welfare stated in the preface that "this document reveals with dramatic clarity that the cigarette is even more dangerous—indeed far more dangerous—than was supposed in 1964."

To be sure, the first warning of the Surgeon General in 1964 did not fall totally on deaf ears. The following fourteen years witnessed a 10 percent decline in the use of cigarettes, as some twenty million smokers stopped or tried to quit. But in 1977 the American public still bought more than 650 billion cigarettes, averaging out over half a pack a day for every person in the country over the age of eighteen. At the present time a full 40 percent of the male and 29 percent of the female population smokes. Especially alarming is the lack of decline in the number of children who smoke.

Thus, anyone who would change the situation has a lot of work cut out for him. But education of the public to the benefits of healthful living, complete banning of cigarette advertisements, elimination of easy availability of cigarettes to young people, halting of government subsidies to tobacco growers, restrictions on smoking in public places, and heavy taxation of cigarettes may partially help improve the situation.

Diet is the second most important environmental factor known to affect numerous cancers. As with smoking, diet, too, is a delicate and highly personal matter, one not easily altered. In 1979 estimated cancers of the five organ sites most related to diet represent a third of all cases. They are cancers of the breast, colon, stomach, esophagus, and the liver and bile ducts.

Breast cancers, the most common form among women (107,000 cases estimated in 1979) appear to be stimulated by high levels of estrogen hormones. Some of the anaerobic microorganisms in the intestine may produce estrogen from normally occurring bile salts. High levels of dietary fats stimulate the production of bile by the liver, as well as increase the proportion of anaerobes in the colon. The body may also manufacture estrogen from stored fat in the adipose tissue. More body mass increases the number of fat cells and thus the amount of estrogen created. Obesity and high levels of dietary fats, therefore, intensify the risk of breast cancer.

Colon cancers are the second most common form of this group, with some 112,000 cases estimated in 1979. Studies have shown that its incidence in various countries correlates closely to the per capita consumption of meat. The greater the amount of meat in the diet, the higher the cancer rate. Several theories have attempted to explain the phenomenon.

First, it takes meat longer to go through the gastrointestinal tract due to its low-fiber content. The longer period gives more time for microorganisms to produce carcinogenic substances from bile salts and other undigested materials. Second, the level of the bacterial enzyme beta glucuronidase is significantly higher in the colon of those on meat-containing diets. Intestinal microorganisms normally secrete the enzyme, but its level fluctuates in individuals according to their diet.

Beta glucuronidase promotes the cleavage of glucuronic acid from other substances. The body normally adds glucuronic acid to potentially harmful substances in the liver as part of the organ's detoxification process. When glucuronic acid is removed in the colon, toxic substances are liberated there, some of which may be carcinogenic. This, coupled with slower transit times of foods through the intestines, can be a dangerous combination.

The causes of gastric cancers (23,000 cases estimated in 1979) are even less understood. Their rates are unusually high in Japan, Chile, Colombia, Austria, Iceland, and Finland. Migration from a high-risk to a low-risk area resulted in a decrease in stomach cancers but an increase in colon cancers. A study conducted in the United States found that stomach-cancer patients ate raw vegetables less often, but it could not determine any relationship between fried foods, meats, or alcohol consumption and the disease. Using more milk, eggs, and dairy products appears to reduce the likelihood of the cancer.

Alcohol consumption and a low intake of vitamins A, C, and riboflavin, as well as the habit of eating steaming-hot food, trigger esophageal cancer (8,000 cases estimated in 1979).

Cancers of the liver and bile duct (11,600 cases estimated in 1979) can result from cirrhosis of the liver brought on by malnutrition or infectious diseases or both. Continuous irritation of the gallbladder by gallstones can lead to cancers of the bile duct. In certain population groups in Africa, South China, Hawaii, and Mozambique, two thirds of all cancers are liver cancers, most likely caused by aflatoxin and other dietary contaminants.

The prudent diet, currently recommended to cut the risk of various cancers, is one low in fat—35 percent or less of the total calorie intake. Even that should consist of a fifty-fifty mixture of polyunsaturated vegetable oil and saturated fats. In addition, physicians recommend a low cholesterol intake of 300 milligrams or less. The diet should also contain liberal amounts of vegetables with high-fiber content and of nonmeat proteins.

A third environmental factor suspected to cause certain cancers is radiation. As a preventive measure, avoiding prolonged exposure to the sun's rays is an obvious but wise step. The deep tan, once the symbol of health, in fact is now a sign of carelessness or ignorance of the dangers of ultraviolet radiation. Likewise, one should seek to minimize exposure to X rays, even for diagnostic purposes.

Another suspected factor is stress. Certain religious groups, such as the Mormons and Seventh-day Adventists, have strikingly lower incidence of cancer even at anatomical sites not generally associated with smoking or alcohol consumption. It seems that a less stressful life-style, a by-product of religious commitment, benefits all parts of the body.

Stress, in experimental animals, raises the level of the hormone corticosterone in the blood and shrinks the lymphatic organs, thymus, lymph nodes, and the spleen. In man, too, such physiological changes could contribute to the growth and proliferation of cancer cells.

Recent studies have implicated the hormone treatments that women have taken for symptoms accompanying the change of life as a possible contributor to cancer of the lining of the uterus, the endometrium. Physicians are advised to prescribe estrogens less frequently and then, in smaller doses for shorter periods of time.

Precancerous changes of the cervical cells generally precede cancer of the cervix. The "Pap smear" test identifies such a development and alerts the physician to the potential danger. Yearly Pap smear tests are recommended. As seen in Table 2, such a practice could forestall about 20 percent of that particular cancer. Herpes virus type II causes blistering of the cervical cells, and the irritations may degenerate into cancerous lesions. Because sexual contact transmits the virus, a promiscuous life-style increases the risk of cervical cancer.

Medical science knows of a number of other pathological conditions that lead to cancer unless they receive proper treatment. They include lumps in the thyroid gland, gallstones, and familial warts in the lower bowel. The proper preventive step in all such cases is surgical removal of the affected parts before they turn cancerous. Sometimes ulcers come into this category as well. A stomach ulcer that does not heal in three months may require an operation.

In summary, we observe that a person's fate as far as contracting various sorts of cancers is concerned, rests to a great measure in his own hands. Life-style and dietary habits contribute measurably to an increased risk of, or protection against, cancer. Currently available knowledge is unequivocal on the factors that enhance cancer: tobacco smoking, consumption of alcohol, a diet high in meat, cholesterol or saturated fat, excess intake of calories in any form, and a stressful or promiscuous life-style. Avoiding them, on the other hand, measurably lowers the risk of cancer.

Chapter 5

The Pound of Cure

The universal cure for cancer is not yet available, and it does not appear that "it is just around the corner." Treatment, however, frequently prolongs the life of the patient many years, sometimes even resulting in complete healing. It represents a significant improvement over that of a typical cancer patient around the turn of the century. At that time few cancer patients could expect to be alive five years from the time of diagnosis. In the 1930s the five-year survival rate was less than 20 percent; in the 1950s, 25 percent; and in the 1970s it reached 30 percent, or approximately one case out of three (see also Table 3).

The main forms of treatment are surgery, radiotherapy, chemotherapy, and immunotherapy. A brief survey of each type follows:

Table 3:

Five-Year Survival Rate

Type of Cancer	1940-1949	1960-1964	1965-1969
Colon	32%	45%	45%
Breast	53%	63%	64%
Cervix	47%	57%	56%
Lung	4%	9%	9%

Because of lack of adequate early-detection techniques, the most common situation the doctor and patient face is one in which the disease is already well-established at the time of diagnosis. The physician's immediate task is to remove the tumor surgically, if the location of the growth permits it. The unequivocal identification of the nature of the tumor rests with the pathologist, who examines its cells under the microscope. If the growth is benign, the surgeon's task is finished. If, however, it is cancerous, he must also remove a wide rim of healthy tissue from the site surrounding the tumor. In general, the smaller the cancerous growth, the more favorable are the chances for the five-year survival (see Table 4).

Table 4:
Relationship Between Five-Year Survival
and Size of Breast Cancer Tumors

Diameter of Tumor	Percent Chance for Five-Year Survival
Less than ¾ inch	76
¾ to 2 inches	55
2 to 4 inches	25

Unfortunately it is not possible to determine whether some of the cancer cells have already left the main tumor and penetrated other body tissues. The general tendency of cancerous growth to metastasize (migrate from one area to another) is what makes it so dangerous. If cancer cells remained localized in a single tumor, surgery in most cases could deal with them. But cancerous growths shed cells, some of which penetrate body cavities and vessels and enter into the bloodstream, the lymphatic system, or the spinal fluid. Through them, cancer cells travel to distant sites in the body. Those surviving the journey establish colonies that eventually result in new growths.

Most tumors release malignant cells into

the lymph or blood continuously as they grow. The hostile environment of the body fluids destroys the overwhelming majority of them. Some, however, manage to adhere to blood platelets or other large structures, forming clumps. The larger the clumps, the more likely they will lodge in a blood capillary, which serves as a haven to the cancer. From there, cancer cells can cross the capillary walls and produce new tumors, using the nutrients in the blood for growth.

Clinical observations show that particular types of primary tumors travel to specific organs. Breast carcinomas tend to spread to the lung or brain. Lung tumors migrate to the brain or to the adrenal glands, and prostate cancers, to the bone. Their special surface properties enable them to bind to selected types of tissues.

When the disease progresses to the point where the surgeon's scalpel is inadequate, the radiologist steps into the picture and also operates, but without the knife. He uses high-energy radiation, which destroys biological matter by damaging the genetic material or by inactivating protein molecules. Unfortunately it is not possible to attack only the cancerous tissue, for healthy cells, too, are inevitably in line of radiation. Normal cells, however, have the ability to repair radiation damage if it is not too severe, whereas cancer cells frequently lack that capacity.

Following irradiation, cell growth stops for a time, then abnormal cell-division patterns lead to the disintegration of numerous cells. Some tissues that normally proliferate rapidly, such as the blood-forming organs of the bone marrow and the intestinal mucosa-forming cells, have the greatest sensitivity to radiation. Thus anemia and intestinal inflammation or even ulcerations can result as an unpleasant side effect. Another difficulty is that sometimes cancer cells will emerge that are more resistant to radiation than healthy ones.

Despite its shortcomings, radiation is an important alternative therapy. Surgical treatment of certain types of cancer such as that of the larynx, for instance, would destroy normal speech. Radiotherapy on the other hand can, under ideal circumstances, stop the growth and preserve the larynx.

Occasionally medical science combines radiotherapy with chemotherapy. Certain substances, such as 5-bromouracil, when assimilated by cancer cells, render them more sensitive to radiation damage. Chemotherapy, the third alternative way to treat cancer, attempts to inhibit cancer by toxic substances.

It is not a very difficult task to find substances that poison cancer cells. The difficulty is to come up with compounds that will destroy only cancer cells. Ordinarily the chemical makeup of healthy and malignant cells resemble each other. What is toxic to one is most often also to the other. Chemotherapy counts on the ability of normal tissue to recover better than the cancer cells from such highly toxic substances.

Since the 1950s the National Cancer Institute has tested more than 300,000 compounds for their effectiveness in fighting cancer. Out of them, forty have showed varying levels of usefulness in chemotherapy.

A few types of cancers respond well to single chemicals. Methotrexate works against uterine choriocarcinoma, and cyclophosphamide combats Burkitt's lymphoma. Usually, however, physicians use a combination of several chemicals.

Chemotherapeutic substances fall into several categories: the antibiotics, the antimitotics (affects the division of the cell's nucleus), the antimetabolites (affects the metabolic process), and the alkylating agents. Most of these hinder the synthesis of nucleic acids or block certain events of cell division. But chemotherapy has two general drawbacks. Strong, unpleasant side effects accompany the drug treatments, and cancer cells frequently develop resistance to the substances.

A nontoxic method does exist to treat certain types of cancer. It exploits a biochemical difference between healthy and some cancer cells. Normal cells can manufacture the amino acid asparagine, while some malignant cells do not, depending, instead, on their environment for it. The enzyme asparaginase, when injected into the blood, destroys all the asparagine there, depriving cancer cells of one of their essential nutrients. Prolonged asparaginase treatment "starves" the cancer cells to death. Certain forms of human leukemia have been successfully treated by this method. Unfortunately few tumors lack the ability to manufacture their own asparagine.

Some cancer cells differ from normal cells in the makeup of their exterior envelope. Our bodies have a surveillance system that monitors the presence of all foreign substances in the body and eliminates them with help from the antibodies and white blood cells. When the body recognizes the cancer cells, with their unique exteriors, as foreign, the immune system will eliminate them. In theory, we could produce vaccines, using the isolated cancer antigens (the unique portions of the cell surface). Such a vaccine would prevent the onset of the type of malignancy from which the antigen originated. In fact, scientists have developed effective anticancer vaccines against Marek's disease and feline leukemia after they isolated the respective viruses that cause the animal cancers.

Researchers have also observed that nonspecific stimulation of the immune system also helps in the fight against cancer. Weakened bacteria of the *Mycobacterium bovis* successfully prevented the transplantation of experimental tumors in animals. Clinical use of the technique, however, has not yet yielded clear-cut results. At present, immunotherapy seems a promising way to combat cancer, but researchers have not yet been able to translate their results into practical therapeutical use.

Scientists have numerous other methods

under investigation. The theory behind one of them is the notion that we might be able to reverse the malignancy of the cancer cell. Under close microscopic scrutiny, cancer cells often appear immature, less than fully developed. Therefore scientists are testing substances that can help cancer cells differentiate into more normal structures. They have already found one such compound. Dimethylformamide, a commonly used organic solvent, slowed down the growth of human colon-cancer cells in tissue cultures. After treatment, the cells appeared more mature under the microscope than previously. Dimethylformamide also inhibited the growth of tumors in mice in preliminary experiments.

In spite of the progress made, we still have much to discover about effectively treating cancer. It is not surprising to see individuals eagerly trying unconventional or controversial methods. But the best chances of recovery still involve cooperating with physicians who have specific training in cancer treatment.

Chapter 6

Living With Cancer

Most of us go through life as if we were immortal. We do not ordinarily pay attention to the fact that every part of our bodies functions properly. Instead we take our good health for granted. Thoughts of death hardly ever enter our minds. In the stories we enjoy most, the ones with happy endings, the hero always lives to the end. And in our personal lives, we are the central character, the "hero." What would become of our story if we were to die?

We are busy living, pursuing our diverse goals, accomplishing what we perceive to be our mission, while the birthdays roll by like numbers on the odometers of cars.

Our culture worships youth, health, and vigor. Each of us wants to be accepted and appreciated, but everyone is getting older. Naturally we cover up as best we can the telltale signs of age. The cosmetic industry offers hundreds of products to help us. When we reach the age of sixty-five or so, however, regardless of how youthful we appear and how much vigor we possess, society often puts us out to pasture through retirement. If we are ailing, we wind up in nursing homes or hospitals. Old and sick people must remain out of sight as much as possible. Otherwise they spoil modern society's pleasant illusion of eternal well-being.

Illness of any sort is a most unwelcome reminder of our frailty. But no sickness comes close to the devastating psychological impact of cancer. In fact, the typical reaction is one of incredulity: "This cannot be happening to me!" Instantly we seem to hear the sentence of death. Our perspective on existence undergoes rapid and drastic revision. The value of time increases immensely while that of objects—"things"— depreciates markedly.

In a private survey by the ABC television company in 1976, Californians confessed to a greater dread of cancer than of being the victims of violent crimes or even of an atomic war.

The diagnosis of cancer suddenly transforms an apparently healthy person to a seriously ill patient. It precipitates anxiety, anger, and grief.

Anxiety differs from fear in that it is a reaction to imagined and anticipated danger and can put more stress on the individual than the illness itself. It has many sources: the specter of death, the effects of medical treatment, the alienation from and abandonment by family and friends.

Anger is also a powerful emotion, whether directed at individuals, situations, or even objects. A cancer patient has a right to be angry—angry at the illness especially. Such an emotion may have a positive, healing effect. On the other hand, if he directs it against physicians, nurses, family members—it can cause alienation, frustration, and hinderance to recovery.

The grief results from sorrow for lost health and lost opportunities (imagined or real), for "life never lived." It helps the patient to be in an environment where he can freely express his grief, for it needs to be shared. Sensitive individuals should enter into grief-sharing sessions with the patient.

The Challenge of Cancer

In view of the serious psychological impact of the discovery of cancer, an important question is: How much should the patient know of his condition? Doctors and family members frequently withhold information from the patient, thinking to spare him undue worry, anxiety, and even depression. But such a tactic usually does not work. Most persons can guess cancer from the nature and extent of treatment prescribed. The majority of individuals want to know the complete truth from their doctors so that they can face the future realistically and get on with the task of coping with cancer.

It is best, also, that the patient knows about the details of the treatments. The physician should take time to explain to him the reasons for surgery, the method, and the expected consequences. Open discussions permit the patient to become an active, rather than passive, participant in the proceedings.

Our culture puts such a high premium on perfection, beauty, strength, and youth that we accept them as the norm, even though most of us do not measure up to such ideals. Surgical treatment for cancer may tempt the patient to devalue himself in comparison with others and withdraw from social contact. He needs reassurance that he is still a valuable member of society.

It is a sad fact that friends and acquaintances frequently shun cancer victims. Uncomfortable in the presence of one whom they perceive to be dying, they don't know what to say and what not to say. Some may even stay away for fear that they will catch the disease. In general they appear to transfer the repulsiveness of cancer to the individual himself. "Visitors always want to hear that I am all right," cancer patients typically comment. "They never have the patience to listen to the whole story of my illness."

Family members may manifest some of the same attitudes. If the cancer patient lives in a family setting, the reactions of family members may materially affect the success or failure of medical treatment. So important is the supportive environment that doctors should study the patient's family situation if he is not making progress during therapy.

It cannot be assumed that the family understands or appreciates the patient's fears. They are likely to be upset. The mounting medical bills, the loss of earning power, and the uncertainty of the future often provoke resentment among the family members. Not uncommonly they hesitate to touch the patient or even his personal belongings. The afflicted one senses their feelings, thus lowering his morale and blunting his response to the medical treatments.

The patient needs supporting, loving relationships, best provided by a husband or a wife or other close family members. It is not realistic, however, to expect individuals to carry such responsibilities single-handedly for extended periods. Friends, neighbors, professional colleagues, fellow church members, must also rally around the stricken family.

If at all possible, definite plans should be laid to rehabilitate the patient to his former role in society. The worst possible strategy is to sit around and wait for something to happen. Idleness at this point is truly demoralizing. One reason for lack of action may be an all-pervading feeling of "What's the use?" Indeed the life of a recuperating former cancer patient does contain many uncertainties. For example, no one can judge his life expectancy or determine what useful active time he has left.

But a return to the world of work brings

emotional relief and financial assistance, one of the primary aims of rehabilitation. Unfortunately, sometimes the employers are reluctant to hire former cancer patients. If the person is disfigured, the employer may consider that it detracts from his business. The possibility of the cancer's recurring may also discourage him.

It should encourage many to know that there are one and a half million Americans living today who are considered cured of cancer. Generally we measure the success of cancer therapy in "five-year survival" times. Actually there is nothing magical about that period. The survival rates could just as well be in terms of four or six years.

Survival times beyond the initial diagnosis does not adequately indicate successful therapy. We must detemine the quality of life, namely, *how* are the patients alive? Are they invalids, depending on others for physical and emotional care? Are they living as recluses, hiding from family and friends? Have they returned to gainful employment and rich personal existence? What is gained if we save large numbers to live in a nightmare?

Unhappily, little study has been done on

how to help those who do survive to have full, productive, satisfying lives. But social scientists have identified several important factors affecting it. These are:

1. The health of the person: Is it abundant or feeble?

2. His functions: Can he carry on personal living chores and work assignments? Can he work as well as he did before the disease?

3. His comfort: Is he free from pain or in frequent distress?

4. His emotional response: Is he able to accept his altered self-image? Is he willing to be reintegrated into his family and community?

5. His financial situation: Does he have sufficient funds for comfortable living, or does he face bankruptcy?

The individuals attempting to show their concern for the cancer patient should keep these factors in mind.

Those classified as "incurable," meaning that current medical science is not equal to the task of curing their cases, form a special category of cancer patients. They have unique needs.

Somehow they need to accept the possibility that their illnesses will recur, but at the same time they also need to maintain hope. "Incurable" and "hopeless" are definitely not synonymous terms. Even if medical science cannot promise a cure, the patient can expect the medical team to control the disease. If they cannot do that, at least he can still hope for comfort.

Those in positions of emotional support need to foster a positive attitude toward life and a will to live. At the same time, however, the cancer victim must come to terms with the intimate and personal meaning of death.

A person with incurable cancer needs the healing power found in crying. Family and friends must help the person express his feelings by being patient listeners. Getting it out in the open frequently benefits the patient.

Persons who have a strong network of close relationships prior to the loss of a loved one can handle grief and mourning easier themselves. In our mobile society close-knit friends and nearby relatives are in short supply.

The cancer victim is concerned about the future welfare of his family after he is gone. Frequently the family itself can work out the problem.

71

One farmer prepared a detailed schedule for the year, in which he wrote in the dates that cotton should be planted, the livestock sold, the wheat sown and harvested, insurance and taxes paid. When he finished the list he carefully went through it, first with his wife, then with their two teenage children. He gained relief from the planning and discussion, and the family successfully lived by that schedule for a number of years.

Putting one's house in order financially and spiritually are urgent problems for many. Individuals in supportive roles can assist by contacting professionals capable of helping—a lawyer for financial planning, a clergyman for spiritual needs.

The incurable cancer patient needs the continual assurance that the medical team handling his case will not give up. Moreover, they must accord him consideration and dignity, to which he is entitled as an important human being.

Perhaps the cancer patient's single most important need is companionship. Waiting for death is the loneliest time for anyone. Such a patient often yearns for the soft touch, the understanding ear, the involvement in family affairs.

Family members often feel that they must keep up a cheerful front regardless of the situation. But the patient may misinterpret this as indifference. It is far better for the family to share their true feelings with him or her. Sharing grief and hope with one another is one of the most rewarding experiences in which a family can participate.

During their trials many terminal cancer patients gain insights that are deep and enriching to those who care to listen. Ruth Burgeson, a professor of English at Walla Walla College for twenty-one years, was one such person. Out of her experience she wrote the following for presentation during a program at the Walla Walla College Church (quoted by permission of the "Walla Walla College Alumni Review").

"Those of you who know me will understand why I am speaking on the subject of living one day at a time, and living that day to the fullest. But since I don't want to speak to anyone in riddles, I'll tell the rest of you why this concept has been especially dear to me for the past four years.

"After being given a diagnosis of cancer,

that at the time of surgery had already spread, I was faced with the hard issue of how to live with the Monster Cancer without being reduced to a sad-faced, fearful, depressed woman from whose life all joy and just plain fun had departed. As I talked with the hospital chaplain on the subject of living under the shadow of death—a conversation, incidentally, that I initiated—one of the most helpful ideas that resulted was not a new one at all, but an old one, hitting my consciousness with a new urgency: Live one day at a time and live that day to the fullest.

"I sometimes think procrastination is one of the greatest of all sins, and how often we confess to it. But how serious is the matter of putting off the business of living, as if we had a thousand years of mortal life! 'When I finish college, then I'll really live.' 'After I'm established in my profession, I'll have time for the things that count.' 'When the children are grown, then I'll have time to do the things that matter.' And decade follows decade and we find we have never really lived.

"A doctor tells of an experience with a forty-five-year-old woman who was dying of cancer. One day he came into her room and found her crying. When he tried to comfort her, she shook her head. 'I'm not crying because I'm going to die,' she said. 'I'm crying because I never really lived.'

"Anyone who has studied T. S. Eliot's poem 'The Love Song of J. Alfred Prufrock' will remember the line where the 'Eternal Footman' holds Prufrock's coat and snickers. If you studied the poem with me, you will probably remember some of our comments on the line as we explored the reason for the snicker of the Eternal Footman, Death, as he holds the coat of one about to depart. The answer of course is to be found in the whole poem, but especially in the lines, 'There will be time—there will be time.' J. Alfred Prufrock was a master of procrastination, putting off the business of living, and Death was gloating over the fact that he was claiming as his a man who had never lived—only existed.

"But I'm wondering about us. Are we living in a land of tomorrows? Or are we savoring each new day as it comes to us? If we can't hike a mountain trail, can we still find majesty and challenge in the foothills? Does the redness of a rose, the call of a meadowlark, the wonder of grass, the miracle of a growing tree, excite us?

Does the smile of a child, the kind deed of a neighbor, the handclasp and understanding of a friend, find a response in our hearts? And as we study and meditate and pray, do we catch new glimpses of what God is like? Do we find companionship with Jesus Christ a reality? Perhaps these are some of the test questions to determine whether we are living each day to the fullest or merely watching the hours pass.

"It was William Allan White (of Emporia, Kansas, fame) who said, 'I am not afraid of *tomorrow*, for I have seen *yesterday*, and I love today.' And I come up with my echo: 'I do not know about tomorrow, but I love today.' And I guess that's about all any of us has."

Chapter 7

The Challenge of Cancer

The ancient Egyptians had a strange custom. Sometimes in the midst of a party, when the celebration reached its peak and the guests were in their most jubilant mood, the host would have a human skull brought out and placed before the celebrants. He did it to heighten his guests' sense of pleasure by reminding them of the transitory nature of existence.

Cancer is the skull on our tables. It bluntly reminds us of our finite status. We begin asking, What is meaningful in our lives? For what do we want to be remembered—and by whom—when we are gone? In short, cancer challenges us to give account of our lives.

Recently I broke a bone above my ankle, and any movement on foot became a painful chore. As I watched the carefree walking of others, I was keenly aware of their gift of the freedom of walking even though they were not. Cancer patients, observing others who are well, are acutely conscious of the apparently abundant gift of time, of which they have so little. To compensate, they learn to handle their time with great care. They find pleasure in ordinary activities, enhancing the quality of their existence.

As perspectives shift under the shadow of cancer, opportunities arise for inner growth. Plans they had held in reserve for the future they now either implement or abandon. They put financial and family obligations in order and face tomorrow with serenity.

Developing a meaningful philosophy of life while battling cancer is no small task, and not all who attempt it succeed. To cope successfully with cancer, it helps to already have a meaningful perspective prior to the onset of the disease.

A deep faith in the Creator and in His constant care is perhaps the most successful of such philosophies. God created a perfect world, we learn from the Scriptures, but man's rebellion against his Maker plunged it into chaos. Cancer and other illnesses dramatically display the world's disorder.

Mankind has not been left alone to suffer the inevitable consequences of his sins. God Himself became the Sin Bearer, accepting the punishment reserved for sinners. To an age-old question—"If God is all powerful, all knowing and abundant in goodness, why did He permit suffering?"—we find the answer on the cross of Calvary. Here we observe the Creator stretched between heaven and earth, voluntarily submitting to one of the cruelest tortures devised by man.

God in Christ voluntarily limited His divine powers and died on the cross for man's sake. Had He not done that, mankind would have perished in its sins.

The believer accepts the sad fact that God continues to limit His powers, permitting the enemy of God and man to bring distress upon us. The assurance that the reign of sin and sickness will not be eternal, that it will come to an abrupt and permanent halt at the second coming of Christ, however, encourages him.

In the meanwhile, believers have a wonderful promise, "We know that in everything God works for good with those who love him"

(Romans 8:28, RSV). Ruth Burgeson, the woman quoted in the previous chapter, comments on the relationship between her religion and her illness:

"I don't believe being a Christian is a guarantee that you won't have these human feelings of sorrow and fear, mental and physical pain, panic—you name it. For me, being a Christian has meant that I didn't have to face these things alone. I believe in a God who cares. That has strengthened me. I expect some day He'll tell me why, but if He told me now, I wouldn't understand it. I am going to let that question rest."

To illustrate the way some Christians have met the challenge of cancer in their lives, I have included two firsthand accounts of battles with the disease. Dr. Ruth Murdoch, professor of education at Andrews University, a well-known and much loved educator, wrote the first one. She has taught almost forty years in the Seventh-day Adventist school system. During this period she has been a strong positive influence in the lives of thousands of young people from elementary through university levels. In recognition of the outstanding contribution she has made to Adventist education, Andrews University named the elementary school it operates in her honor in 1976.

"It had been an unusually busy summer," she wrote, "as I had been teaching summer school, gathering data for my dissertation; and making preparation for a move from Takoma Park, Maryland, to the campus of Emmanuel Missionary College, in Michigan. That morning we had seen our furniture and household goods loaded into the van and started on the two-day trip across country. In the late afternoon we finished the final cleaning of the house and left in the car, expecting to spend the night in a motel and then overtake the van so we could arrive ahead of it to see our goods unloaded.

"That night in the motel after my husband and ten-year-old son had retired, I was brushing my hair when I discovered a lump in my right breast. For a few moments I was seized with real panic because cancer had been common in my family and I knew the possibilities involved. I glanced in the mirror and noticed that my face had broken out with a cold sweat. My first impulse was to awaken my husband and suggest that we return to Takoma Park, where I knew that we had a hospital and I was acquainted with the doctors. However, I realized there was not that urgency and if I were to awaken him at that time he probably would not rest much the remainder of the night. I looked across the room at our sleeping son, realizing that the next years ahead of him were so vital to his development, and I thought of the possibility that I would not be there to guide him. Then my faith grasped some of God's promises. I got my Bible and read for a little while, then went over and knelt by the child's bed and committed him to the care of our heavenly Father, knowing that my life was in God's hand and that He could heal me and give the doctors success if this was His will. I was then able to retire and sleep comfortably all night. The next morning the sun was so bright and lovely, the fall so beautiful, that it didn't seem the time to suggest a return to Washington, so we continued our journey and arrived at Berrien Springs that night.

"The next morning I told my husband I felt I should get in touch with a doctor in the Berrien Springs area. He quickly reminded me that the doctor whom we had entertained in England during the war years was a very successful surgeon in nearby Niles. I called his sister and found that he had been on vacation and was returning the same afternoon. She agreed to talk with her brother, the doctor, and a few hours later called to say that he was heavily booked with surgery for the next month or more but that he would come into the office a day early if need be. An appointment was made for the following Sunday afternoon.

"At the time of the first examination the doctor said quietly, 'I wish I could tell you that I think it is only an enlarged gland, but all the characteristics of a malignancy are present.' He then said that I should come into the hospital on Monday afternoon and that the surgery would be scheduled for Tuesday morning. He also said that if the biopsy revealed no abnormal cells, they would remove only the enlarged gland and that I would know when I came out from the anesthetic because my arm would be free and able to move.

"As arranged, I entered the hospital on Monday evening. After the nurse had made me comfortable, she brought me a tablet and asked me to take it, saying that the doctor wanted to be sure I had a good night's rest. I told her that I did not usually need any help in going to sleep and that if it was agreeable with her I would rather leave the tablet on the table, and then if I was not asleep by 9:30 or 10:00, I would be glad to take it. She called the doctor and he agreed to this arrangement. The next morning the nurse told me that she came in twenty minutes later and I was fast asleep. The night nurse recorded that I had slept well all night. This of course helped me to awaken with courage and confidence on Tuesday morning. When I came out from under the effects of the anesthetic I discovered that my arm was tightly bandaged down my side, so I did not need to ask whether or not it was malignant.

"A few days later when I was to be released from the hospital the doctor told me that he would recommend forty-five X-ray treatments as a precautionary measure in case there might have been some spreading that had not been detected. He said that the X rays would be somewhat unpleasant, that I would suffer from what would appear to be a severe sunburn, and that I would also experience some nausea. The X-ray treatments lasted until Thanksgiving. However, I was able to begin my teaching on the new campus two weeks after the surgery. I took back one class at a time until within ten days I was carrying my full load. Fortunately, my classes came in the afternoon, and since the X-ray treatments were in the morning, I was able to rest a little bit afterward. To my surprise I discovered that when I got in the classroom and involved with teaching, the extreme feelings of nausea disappeared.

"Naturally, there were many thoughts that went through my mind and snatches of poetry concerning death seemed to reoccur in my mind many times. However, whenever these thoughts of depression came I again committed my life to the Lord and told Him that if it was His will that I should live and continue taking care of my family, rearing our youngest son and teaching classes, that I would devote my entire life to His service. I decided that I would never refuse any opportunity to witness for Him.

"Soon the question came to my mind as to whether or not I should go ahead and finish the dissertation. I had already written four of the seven chapters, but I was not sure whether, under the circumstances, this was the way I should spend my time. Then realizing that I had asked the Lord for His blessing and health and an extension of time, I concluded that if I had real faith I would go ahead and finish the task. Soon after Thanksgiving I got out my manuscripts and spent Saturday nights and what time I could spare from my other duties to finish the work on the dissertation. It was completed before spring, and in June of 1960 the degree was conferred. That was twenty years ago.

"There were five of us who went to the hospital for X rays at the same time. Today I am the only one of the five who is still alive and enjoying good health. For this I continue to thank the Lord. Once again I dedicate the time that He gives me to His service, hoping to be a blessing to others and share the story of His love."

Gordon Dalrymple, an evangelist, pastor, editor, and director of public relations for the television program, "Faith for Today," and later for the radio program, "Voice of Prophecy," wrote the second narrative:

"Cancer! It had always been a scare word to me.

"One night while traveling in Florida I noticed a small spot of blood and a discharge on the back of my shirt.

" 'The heat,' I said to myself as I thought of Florida's humidity.

"Arriving home, I was caught short by my wife's startled exclamation over the growth on my back. I had almost forgotten it.

" 'Better get to a doctor right away,' Lois suggested. 'It might be something serious.'

"In my lifetime I had known almost no illness. I was inclined to dismiss the spot on my back. It might simply go away.

"But later that day, prompted by the urgings of Lois and a momentary apprehension of my own, I was in the doctor's office. He suggested an immediate biopsy.

"The surgeon doubted there was anything malignant in the sore. But he removed a wide enough area so that if there was anything malignant it would be removed. Nothing like playing it safe.

"When I returned three days later, the surgeon announced, 'It's malignant. It's melanoma.' Melanoma, he explained, was one of the deadliest and fastest growing of the cancers. It hopscotches around the body, growing where it chooses.

"But caught early, melanoma can be removed easily. No danger when the infected part of the body is removed. By going deep enough and wide enough, the cancer can be stopped before it spreads through the body.

"A person does not have a good part of his back cut away without asking questions.

" 'Is surgery absolutely necessary?' I asked.

" 'Listen,' the doctor explained patiently. 'I had a friend who had melanoma and died from it in six weeks in spite of all we could do. If *I* had melanoma, *I* would have a cut made as deep and as wide as possible.'

"His earnestness was convincing.

"The surgery, which was done under a local anesthetic, went smoothly. No, the surgeon said, there was no way to be sure that all the melanoma was being removed. But there were no indications melanoma existed anywhere else in my body. And there were numerous cases of melanoma being stopped by early surgery. We would hope this would happen in my case.

"The round of quarterly checkups revealed nothing—for about a year. But the fourth checkup indicated that the melanoma might have recurred.

"Three biopsies were ordered in separate

locations on my back. Two were negative; the other revealed recurring melanoma, and a careful check under the right arm showed one enlarged lymph node—probably invaded by melanoma.

"This time surgery would have to be far more drastic. A large section of my back would be cut away, and the lymph nodes would be removed under both arms.

"December 4, 1974, I checked into the hospital. That was the exact date I was to begin a short series of evangelistic meetings in Chattanooga, Tennessee. I had asked the doctors for a five-day delay so I could conduct the series. But in dealing with melanoma, time is of the essence. A few days could mean the difference.

"When I awoke in the recovery room the doctor explained that the enlarged lymph node had been invaded by melanoma. 'I should tell you,' he said calmly, professionally, 'your chances of living more than five years are slightly less than 50 percent. But we will do all we can. As soon as you are out of the hospital, we will try immunotherapy.'

"The treatments went well—for a few weeks.

"Then one day in my office at the Voice of Prophecy a sudden pain struck the back of my head, rolled across my forehead, and ended in my right eyeball. It was the first headache of my life. I had never before taken even an aspirin. I went for a drink of water. When I returned, the pain in my head came back again—this time with a more acute penetrating force. Nausea followed.

"The doctor suggested I enter the hospital. Tests there showed quite plainly that the left side of my body was not as strong as the right. I had known something was wrong two days before when my left foot would not go into a slip-on shoe. At times my left leg through my pelvic region would go to sleep.

"The tests pointed unquestionably to a brain tumor. It was hard to accept the evidence. Finally a brain scan was taken. After several inconclusive tests, the last revealed two small tumors on the right side of the brain.

"Brain cancer! The news could hardly have been worse. When the doctor gave me four weeks to live, I felt a knot of fear in my stomach. The picture was grim. There was no escaping its reality.

"The psychology of fear—I now knew what

it was. As a minister I had visited cancer patients who had simply given up, resigning themselves to death. And I had also known of those who had met the cancer menace courageously and yet had been taken by death.

"Fear at any level of life takes its toll. It can be particularly dangerous when one is facing a scourge like cancer. For the will to live, the mental attitude is crucial. It can mean the difference between life and death.

"A steroid drug, decadron, was used to shrink my brain tumors. Radiation followed. During radiation therapy, which continued for five and one-half weeks, I was not able to drive.

"I could give up and go to bed during the time the radiation treatments were given. Or I could carry on with as near normal a routine as possible.

"Overcoming fear. How important! I remembered the words of a courageous U.S. President, 'Nothing to fear but fear itself.' In my heart I knew that fear could deprive me of my self-confidence, my will to live, my determination to cooperate with doctors and defeat the melanoma—if, indeed, it could be conquered.

"Then the words came to me: 'Fear thou not; for I am with thee' (Isaiah 41:10). 'I will never leave thee, nor forsake thee' (Hebrews 13:5).

"The conviction came that God has the power to heal. When a man has done his best and fails, Heaven can intervene. A great peace swept over me. And I determined I would not yield to blind, unreasoning fear that could defeat me just as surely as melanoma. Regardless of whether it was win, lose, or draw in the contest ahead, I had this mighty Bible promise: 'Yea, though I walk through the valley of the shadow of death, I will fear no evil: for thou art with me' (Psalm 23:4).

"This was the promise I could cherish. With it I could overcome fear and self-pity.

"I also knew God had the power to heal me. This assurance meant far more than radiation, surgery, or any other technique known to man. I recognized that God could heal me instantly, or He could do it through advancing medical science.

"I sensed that there was tremendous power in prayer. And I decided to avail myself of it, requesting but not demanding healing. The precious promises of Scripture swept away all fear.

" 'God is our refuge and strength, a very present help in trouble' (Psalm 46:1). 'Thou wilt keep him in perfect peace, whose mind is stayed on thee: because he trusteth in thee' (Isaiah 26:3). 'Fear thou not; for I am with thee: be not dismayed; for I am thy God: I will strengthen thee' (Isaiah 41:10).

"My wife had asked the doctor about calling in the elders for special prayer. He felt it would be wise. All across the country prayer groups got together—friends, fellow ministers, individuals who had attended meetings I conducted. At my bedside Dr. H. M. S. Richards and his son, H. M. S. Richards, Jr., earnestly asked God to heal me if it was His will. His power, after all, is unlimited.

"The radiation treatments were hardly over (successfully so far as we could tell) when the melanoma struck in the abdomen. A malignant tumor was found there the size of a grapefruit. The doctors were successful in removing a smaller one, but the larger they were afraid to touch. To remove it the surgeon would have to cut across a tumor, releasing an untold number of malignant cells throughout my body. The melanoma was obviously hopscotching throughout my body, striking where it chose.

"I was content to put myself in God's hands. He knew the way. I would not *demand* that He heal. My life had been one full of opportunity. I had come to treasure every moment of it.

"If it were God's plan that I lay it down, well and good. On the other hand, if He were willing for me to have a few more years in which to serve Him, I would rejoice. The fact was, I was in love with my family. And the evangelism and editorial work I was in I enjoyed immeasurably.

"I was glad for the sure promises of God. There could have been craven surrender to fear and the impulses associated with it. But not with the bedrock of God's promises of love and care. They meant everything to me.

"A new chapter of life opened before me. And it was to be written in faith, not fear."

Not long after writing these lines, Pastor Dalrymple passed away. Forty-four years old at the time of his death, he had served his church devotedly throughout his adult life for twenty-four years. In his eulogy Dr. William Fagal, his colleague at Faith for Today, said, "I do not recall anyone in the world who exceeded or even duplicated his Christian courage. He never seemed downhearted and never yielded to discouragement."

God desires to have followers who love Him more than life itself. From time to time He permits the death of a child of His as a demonstration of the meaning of true devotion. But death in the Lord is a mere sleep, a transitory "holding pattern" between this life and the eternal one to come. When cancer strikes the Christian he can say, " 'O death, where is thy sting? O grave, where is thy victory?' " (1 Corinthians 15:55) and will face its menace unafraid.

Indeed to answer the question of Jeremiah 8:22 there is a balm in Gilead; there is a Physician there. The balm is available to all for the asking and so are the services of the Physician. The balm is the solemn promise of the living God, that though we walk through the valley of death, the Physician will be with us till time ends.

Bibliography

Books

Berglass, A. *Cancer: Nature, Cause and Cure.* Inst. Pasteur, 1957.

Bodansky, O. *Biochemistry of Human Cancer.* Academic Press, 1975.

Braun, A. C. *The Cancer Problem.* Columbia U. Press, 1969.

Cairns, J. *Cancer—Science and Society.* Freeman, 1978.

Cantor, R. C. *And a Time to Live.* Harper and Row, 1978.

Hardy, R. E. and J. G. Cull. *Counseling and Rehabilitating the Cancer Patient.* Charles Thomas, 1975.

Harris, R. J. C., ed. *What We Know About Cancer.* St. Martin's Press, 1970.

Hiatt, H. H., J. D. Watson, J. A. Winstein, eds. *Origins of Human Cancer.* Cold Spring Harbor Laboratory, 1977.

Homburger, F., ed. *The Physiopathology of Cancer.* S. Karger, 1974.

Nieburgs, H. E., ed. *Prevention and Detection of Cancer.* Marcel Dekker, Inc., 1978.

Pierce, G. B., R. Shikes, L. M. Fink. *Cancer, a Problem of Developmental Biology.* Prentice-Hall, Inc., 1978.

Periodical Articles

Arcos, J. C. "Cancer: Chemical Factors in the Environment." *American Laboratory,* June, 1978, p. 65, and July, 1978, p. 29.

Burgeson, R. C. "One Day at a Time." Walla Walla College "Alumni Review," Fall, 1978, p. 6.

Cairns, J. "The Cancer Problem." *Scientific American,* November, 1975, p. 64.

Dalrymple, G. "I Will Fear No Evil." Voice of Prophecy *News,* April, 1976, p. 3.

Maugh, T. H. "Chemical Carcinogens: the Scientific Basis for Regulation." *Science 201,* 1978, p. 1200.

_____"Chemical Carcinogens: How Dangerous Are Low Doses?" *Science 202,* 1978, p. 37.

Nicolson, G. L. "Cancer Metastasis." *Scientific American,* March, 1979, p. 66.

Rose, D. P. "Diet, Nutrition, and Cancer." *Life and Health* (cancer prevention special issue), 1978, p. 7.